MW00513580

BRAIN
HEALTH
COOKBOOK

The Tastiest and Quickest Recipes to
Boost Your Mind's Performance

Jamie The Fork

TABLE OF CONTENTS

INTRODUCTION

Alzheimer's disease is a term we've all heard before. Most of us believe it exclusively affects the elderly, and that they lose their memories as a result. But things aren't quite as they seem. It is difficult for the patient, much alone their family, to accept a diagnosis of Alzheimer's disease or dementia.

Alzheimer's disease is the most prevalent type of dementia, which is a brain ailment that has a daily influence on a person's life. Memory loss and cognitive abnormalities are common symptoms. According to the Alzheimer's Association, not all memory loss is caused by Alzheimer's disease. Alzheimer's disease affects one out of every 10 persons over the age of 65, and almost one-third of those over the age of 85.

The symptoms of this condition appear gradually and frequently worsen as time passes. Things may begin with gradual amnesia, which can lead to broad brain damage. This occurs when essential cells die, resulting in severe personality loss and bodily system collapse.

Alzheimer's disease is impossible to diagnose on your own. Make an appointment with your doctor if you feel you or a loved one has it (signs grow more and more visible). Even if you are afraid, early diagnosis and treatment will help you delay the most debilitating symptoms.

You may extend your independence and make the most of your life by using the right medications.

Even though Alzheimer's disease is frequent and older individuals aren't immune to it, there are ways to avoid it. The first step is to make dietary and behavioral changes.

Many individuals are unaware that the food they consume and the manner they spend their life have long-term consequences for their health (even if they are perfectly healthy in the present moment).

Many features of the Mediterranean diet and the DASH (Dietary Approaches to Stop Hypertension) diet are incorporated into the Brain Health Diet. MIND (Mediterranean-DASH Intervention for Neurodegenerative Delay) is a combination of the two terms.) The Brain Health Diet varies from other programs in several key areas, and it has been shown to be more beneficial than both in terms of lowering the risk of Alzheimer's disease.

The goal of this diet is to teach you how to avoid Alzheimer's disease and dementia by modifying your diet and lifestyle. In all aspect of life, information is essential. The sooner you have the necessary information, the sooner you may begin taking action and avoid more damage.

It's never too early to make positive changes in your life and form healthy habits that might preserve your life and allow you to enjoy your latter years in peace.

The beauty of this diet is that it emphasizes eating entire foods. In this diet, processed foods have no place. Fruits, vegetables, olive oil, seafood, nuts, and moderate wine consumption are just a few of the foods available in this diet.

On the other hand, this diet advises against eating red meat and processed foods. Red meats aren't necessarily bad, but for your good health, moderation is important. Also, the longer you cook your meat, the worse for you it becomes.

In brief, eating only lean protein is not good for your health. The Brain Health Diet advises against eating too much meat, especially cooked to a well done stage.

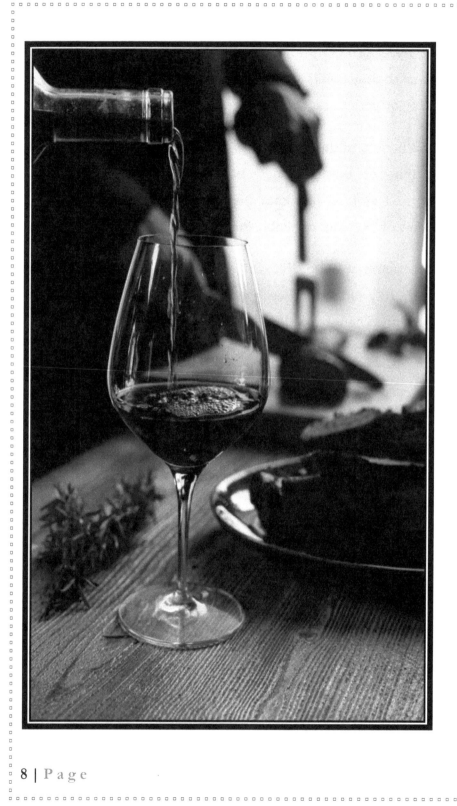

BREAKFAST

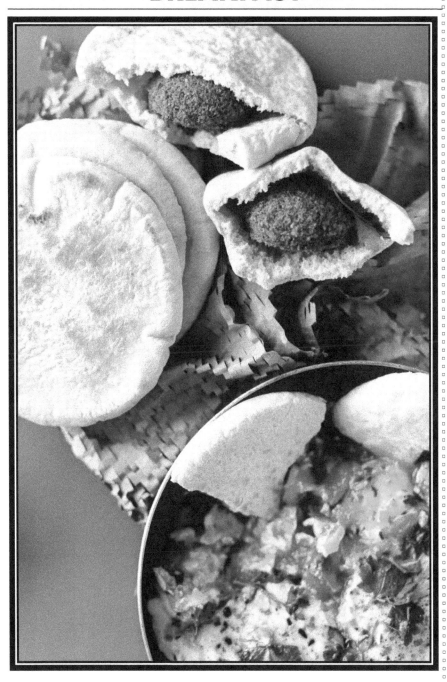

1. DELICIOUS BANANA BUTTERMILK PANCAKES

Servings: 4

Cooking Time: 30 Minutes

Calories: 500

INGREDIENTS:

- Two mugs of low-fat buttermilk

- Half mug egg substitute

- One mug mashed ripened banana

- Two mugs whole grain pastry flour one tsp. baking powder

- One-fourth tsp. baking soda

- One-fourth tsp. salt

- Canola oil cooking drizzle

- Sliced banana or sugar-free or low-sugar fruit jams as garnish

- Sugar-free nectar

INSTRUCTIONS:

1. During a mixing dish, mix flour, baking powder, baking soda, and salt, then build a well in the middle of the batter. In a separate dish, merge the buttermilk and egg and mix to mix. Put buttermilk batter into well and fold in the flour with a spatula until the batter is glossy. Gently fold in banana and permit batter to stand for five minutes. In the meantime, drizzle a skillet with cooking oil and temperature over moderate temperature. Drop some droplets of water onto the heated griddle.

2. When water droplets bead, the grill is warm enough. Put two tbsp. Of batter onto griddle for every pancake. Prepare pancakes until the surface of the pancake begins to bubble, and the perimeters flip golden brown (about three minutes). Flip the pancake over and prepare till the other side is golden brown.

3. Repeat this process till all the batter is gone. Keep cooked pancakes on a warm platter or in a very low-temperature oven (175 degrees) while getting ready for the other pancakes. Serve heat, garnished with diced banana, low-sugar fruit jam, or sugar-free nectar, if need.

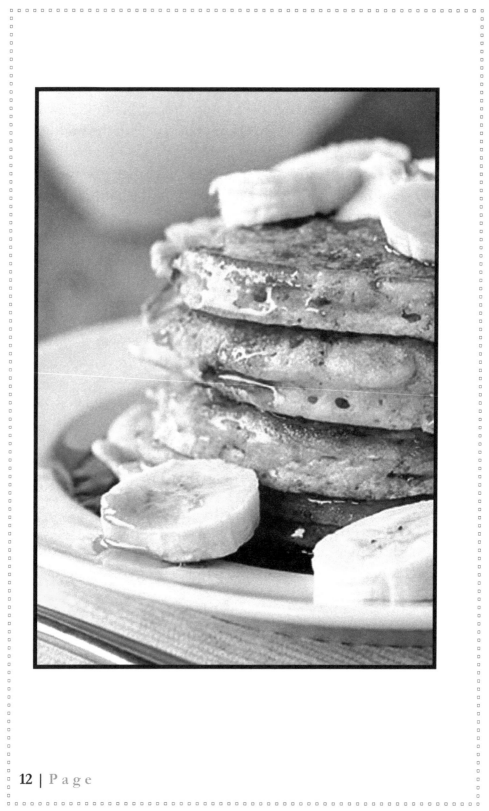

2. GLUTEN-FREE BAKED APPLE PANCAKES

Servings: 2

Cooking Time: 20 Minutes

Calories: 500

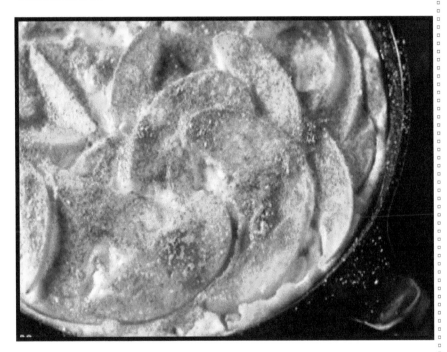

INGREDIENTS:

- One mug flour
- Three tbsp. sugar
- One mug one% milk
- Two egg whites
- Two eggs

- One tbsp. butter
- Four moderate tart apples, peeled and diced
- Three tbsp. Brown sugar
- Half tsp. cinnamon
- Two tsp. vanilla
- Three tbsp. powdered sugar

INSTRUCTIONS:

1. Warm up the oven to 425 degrees Fahrenheit. In a big ovenproof frying pan, melt butter over moderate temperature. Put apples into the pan and drizzle with brown sugar. Prepare, frequently moving, until apples are soft, about 12 to 15 minutes. Drizzle apples with cinnamon and take out from the temperature.

2. Meanwhile, in a moderate-size dish, merge flour and sugar. Put milk, egg whites, eggs, and vanilla and beat just until glossy. Put over apples in a frying pan. Put the pan in oven and oven for 20 minutes. Decrease temperature to 350 degrees Fahrenheit and oven for 12 to 18 minutes longer or until pancake is golden brown. Drizzle with powdered sugar and serve right away.

3. Amazing Cheesy Apple Raisin Cinnamon Omelet

Servings: 3

Cooking Time: 30 Minutes

Calories: 500

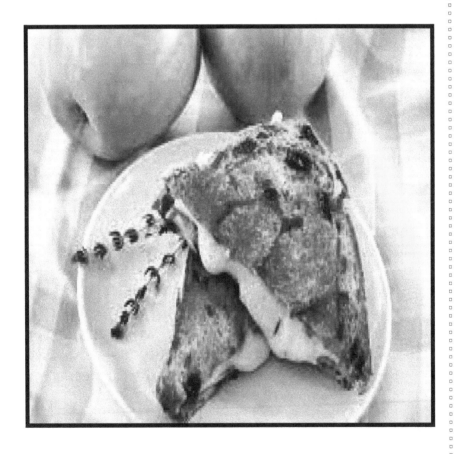

INGREDIENTS:

- One mug of egg whites or four whole eggs
- Two tbsp. cut down into pieces blue cheddar cheese
- Two tbsp. Freshly shredded Parmesan cheddar cheese
- One moderate sweet apple peeled, cored, and diced
- One tbsp. Extra-virgin olive oil
- Two tbsp. seedless black
- Salt and freshly ground pepper to taste
- One-eighth tsp. cinnamon

INSTRUCTIONS:

1. Fry apple slices in half tbsp. Of olive oil until crispy tender; add raisins, then immediately remove apple batter from pan and transfer to a dish.

2. Merge eggs, cheeses, and salt and pepper, and Merge well. Warm-up remaining olive oil in an omelet pan; prepare one-fourth of egg batter simultaneously, on low temperature, lifting edges to permit uncooked portion to flow below and prepare. Repeat the method four times for every serving.

3. Organize one-fourth apple batter onto one-half of the cooked egg. Fold in half and drizzle prime with cinnamon. Serve as a breakfast omelet or a dessert.

4. POACHED EGGS IN A GARDEN

Servings: 2

Cooking Time: 15 Minutes

Calories: 500

INGREDIENTS:

- One moderate red bell pepper, chopped
- One moderate white onion, chopped
- Two mugs button mushrooms, diced
- Two tbsp. olive oil
- Two big russet potatoes, diced
- Two mugs fresh broccoli florets
- Salt and freshly ground pepper to taste eight big eggs, poached

INSTRUCTIONS:

1. Warm the olive oil in a large frying pan over moderately high heat. Place the potatoes, broccoli, red bell pepper, onion, mushrooms, salt, and pepper to taste in a large mixing dish.

2. Cook, sometimes stirring, until the vegetables are tender and the potatoes begin to brown. Serve by dividing the batter into four parts and topping each with two poached eggs.

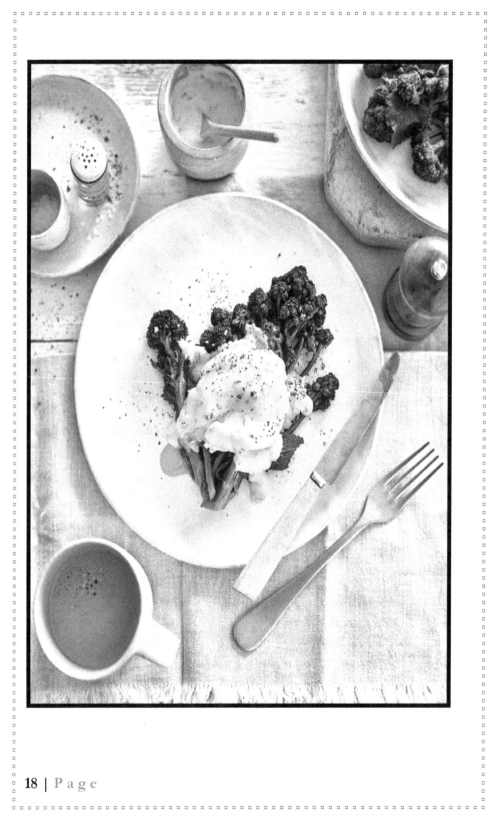

5. GLUTEN-FREE SPANISH OMELET

Servings: 4

Cooking Time: 20 Minutes

Calories: 500

INGREDIENTS:

- Two tbsp. Extra-virgin olive oil
- Six whole scallions,
- Four cloves fresh garlic, thinly diced
- One green bell pepper, seeded and thinly
- Diced one red bell pepper,
- Three ripened tomatoes, peeled and cut into wedges
- Four tbsp. chopped fresh parsley
- Three mugs egg substitute or three mugs egg
- Whites or 12 big eggs
- One-fourth lb. cut down into pieces
- Fresh low-fat goat cheddar cheese
- Salt and freshly ground pepper to taste
- One-fourth tsp. Cayenne pepper
- Third-fourth tsp. Ground cumin
- Half tsp. Ground coriander
- Half tsp. ground cinnamon

INSTRUCTIONS:

1. Heat a pair of tbsp. Olive oil in an oven-safe frying pan and gently fry scallions and garlic for concerning five minutes, till they begin to soften. Put the inexperienced, red bell peppers, zucchini, and tomatoes raise the temperature slightly and continue sautéing another five-15 minute until the vegetables have softened and most of the juice is absorbed. Put salt and pepper to style. Set aside at area temperature.

2. In a huge dish, merge the herbs with the eggs and Merge with a fork simply to interrupt the yolks. Lift the vegetables out of the frying pan with a slotted spoon and merge with eggs. Return the frying pan to moderate temperature, adding more olive oil if necessary.

3. When the olive oil is heat, add the eggs and vegetable batter and prepare for two-three minutes, lifting the edges with a spatula to allow uncooked eggs to run below cooked ones. Crumble goat cheddar cheese over the high of the omelet and transfer frying pan to a four-hundred-degree oven to finish cooking for regarding 15-20 minutes or till omelet is set and therefore the cheddar cheese is melted. It can additionally be served as a lightweight supper.

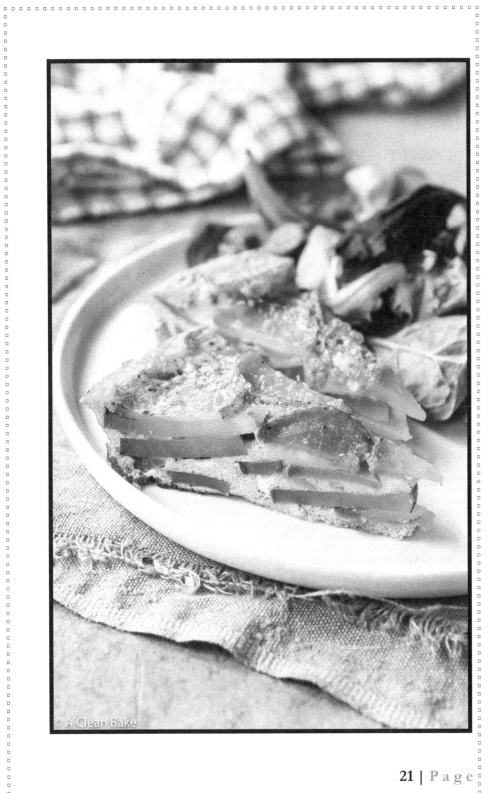

© A Clean Bake

6. STRAWBERRY BUTTERMILK PANCAKES

Servings: 3

Cooking Time: 30 Minutes

Calories: 500

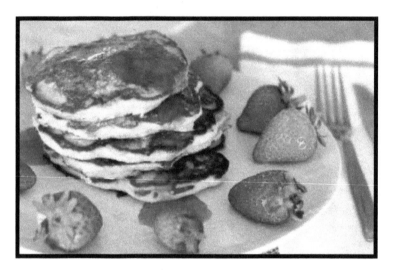

INGREDIENTS:

- One-fourth tsp. salt
- Two mugs of low-fat buttermilk
- Half mug egg substitute
- Two mugs whole grain pastry flour
- One tsp. Baking powder
- One-fourth tsp. Baking soda
- One mug diced fresh strawberries

INSTRUCTIONS:

1. Sliced strawberries or other fruit or low-sugar fruit jams as garnish Sugar-free nectar During a mixing dish, blend along with flour, baking powder, baking soda, and salt, then make a well in the middle of the batter.

2. In a separate dish, merge the buttermilk and egg and mix to mix. Put buttermilk batter into the well and fold in the flour with a spatula until batter is swish. Gently fold in strawberries and allow the batter to square for five minutes.

3. In the meantime, drizzle a skillet with cooking oil and temperature over moderate temperature. Drop a few droplets of water onto the heated griddle. When water droplets bead, the grill is heating enough. Put two tbsp.

4. Of batter onto griddle for each pancake. Prepare pancakes until the surface of the pancake begins to bubble, and the perimeters flip golden brown (about three minutes). Flip the pancake over and prepare until different aspect is golden brown.

5. Repeat this process until all the batter is gone. Keep cooked pancakes on a heated platter or during a low-temperature oven (one hundred seventy-five degrees), whereas getting ready the other pancakes. Serve warm, garnished with diced strawberries, low-sugar fruit jam, or sugar-free nectar, if need

7. Low Carb Broccoli And Cheese Frittata

Servings: 5

Cooking Time: 20 Minutes

Calories: 500

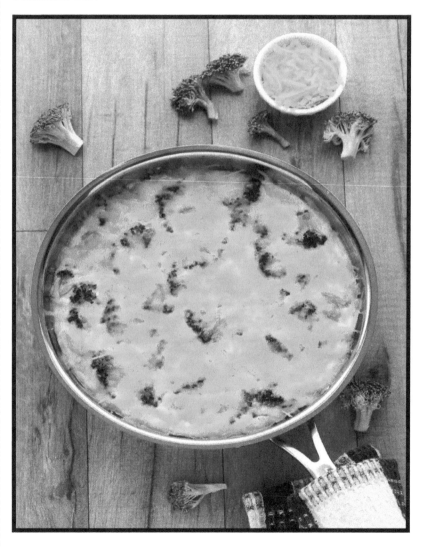

INGREDIENTS:

- Two cloves fresh garlic, minced
- One mug of shredded mozzarella cheddar cheese
- Dash of crushed red, warm pepper flakes
- Three mugs broccoli florets
- One tbsp. Extra-virgin olive oil half mug finely chopped onion
- Half mug chopped red bell pepper
- One half mugs egg substitute or one-half mugs egg
- Whites or six big eggs Olive oil drizzle

INSTRUCTIONS:

1. Steam broccoli until crispy, tender, and remove from temperature. A very massive frying pan over moderate-heat, temperature olive oil and fry onion, bell pepper, and garlic until vegetables are soft (concerning five minutes).

2. Put broccoli and prepare about two minutes longer. Transfer vegetable batter to a dish, then add mozzarella cheddar cheese and heat pepper flakes.

3. If using whole eggs, beat in a separate dish till blended. Beat eggs into vegetable batter and place into a round cake pan lightly sprayed with olive oil drizzle. Oven in a 325-degree oven till eggs are set for thirty minutes. Serve heat or at room temperature.

8. Ham And Zucchini Frittata

Servings: 3

Cooking Time: 30 Minutes

Calories: 500

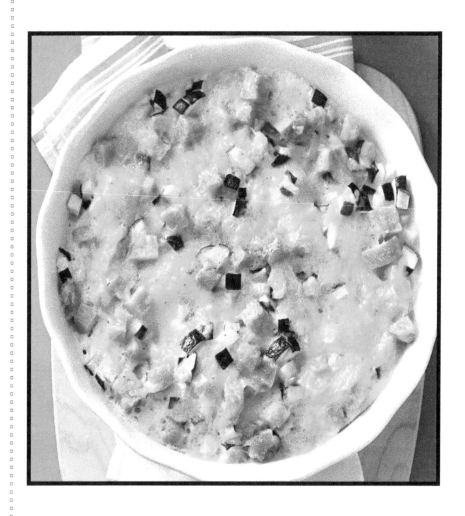

INGREDIENTS:

- One tbsp. olive oil
- One moderate white onion, chopped
- One clove of fresh garlic, minced
- One moderate zucchini,
- Low-sodium ham
- One half mug liquid egg
- One-fourth mug low-fat milk
- One tsp. dry Italian seasoning
- Two Italian plum tomatoes, diced
- One mug shredded, part-skim milk mozzarella cheddar cheese

INSTRUCTIONS:

1. Warm up the oven to grill. In an oven-safe frying pan, temperature olive oil over moderate temperature. Put onion, garlic, and zucchini, fry till soft. Decrease temperature to moderate-low, add ham and prepare for about two minutes.

2. In a dish, merge liquid eggs, milk, Italian seasoning Merge, and salt and pepper to style. Put batter into the frying pan with ham and prepare unstirred for about five minutes or until eggs begin to set.

3. Organize tomato slices on prime of egg batter and drizzle with mozzarella cheddar cheese. Put frying pan about six inches underneath broiler and grill for concerning four-five minutes until eggs are set, and cheddar cheese is gently baked. Drizzle top of the frittata with a touch of Italian seasoning. Merge and serve.

9. Fat-Free Quinoa And Raisins Porridge

Servings: 1

Cooking Time: 20 Minutes

Calories: 500

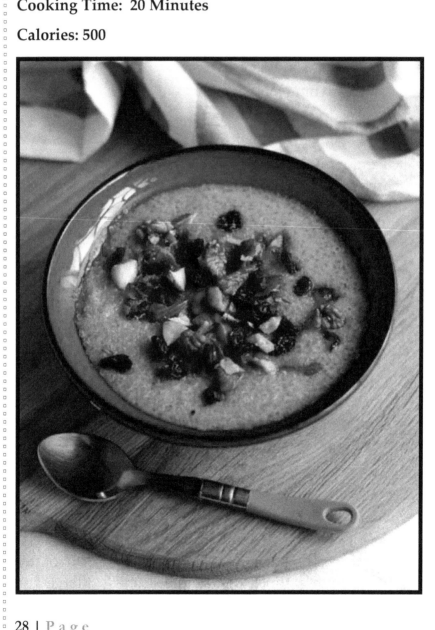

INGREDIENTS:

- One-eighth tsp. Ground nutmeg
- One-eighth tsp. ground ginger
- Dash of salt
- Two tbsp. Pure maple nectar
- Two mugs of almond milk
- One mug quinoa rinsed through a fine-mesh sieve under cold water
- Half tsp. Ground cinnamon
- Half tsp. Pure vanilla essence
- Two tbsp. raisins
- One-fourth mug chopped nuts

INSTRUCTIONS:

1. In a pan over moderate temperature, gently temperature almond milk, moving sometimes until it begins to bubble. Decrease temperature to a stew and add in quinoa, cinnamon, nutmeg, ginger, and salt.

2. Prepare uncovered, sometimes moving, until quinoa is tender and thickens (about 20–25 minutes). Take out from temperature, add in maple nectar, vanilla essence, and raisins. Wrap with a sprinkling of nuts and serve.

10. ZUCCHINI FRITTATA

Servings: 2

Cooking Time: 18 Minutes

Calories: 500

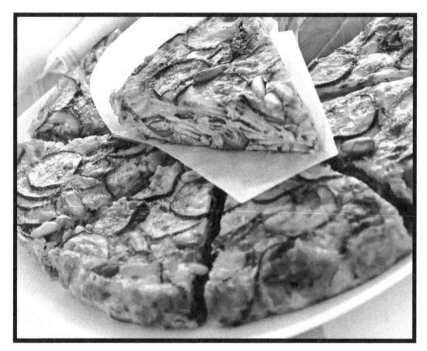

INGREDIENTS:

- Three little zucchinis, diced one-fourth-inch thick
- Freshly ground pepper to taste
- Two tbsp. minced fresh basil leaves
- One-half tbsp. Extra-virgin olive oil, one moderate yellow onion, chopped
- Two cloves fresh garlic, minced

INSTRUCTIONS:

1. In a frying pan over moderate-low temperature, temperature olive oil and fry onion and garlic till soft and gently baked. Place zucchini and salt and pepper to onion garlic batter and prepare another five-eight minute.

2. Take out from temperature and set aside. In a dish, add basil and eggs (beat eggs if using whole eggs) to zucchini batter. Beat batter to mix and place egg batter into a gently greased round cake pan.

3. Oven in the oven at 325 degrees until eggs set. Take out from the oven, drizzle Parmesan cheddar cheese over high frittata, and place beneath the broiler for two-three minutes till cheddar cheese is golden brown. Take out from the oven and serve instantly. It can be served as a lightweight supper.

11. Mexican Avocado and Ham Omelet

Servings: 3

Cooking Time: 25 Minutes

Calories: 500

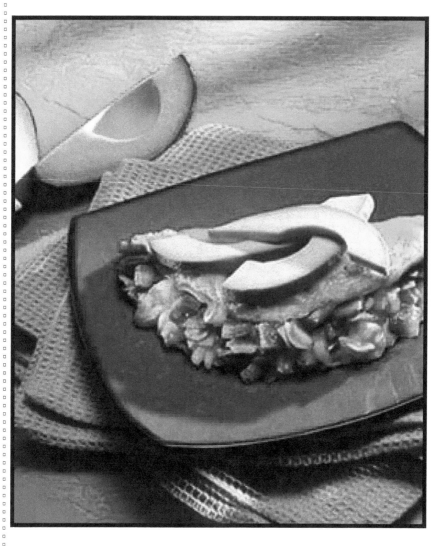

INGREDIENTS:

- One pinch paprika
- One-fourth tsp. salt
- Two tbsp. (30 grams) sour cream
- Two eggs
- One-fourth mug (30 grams) ham, minced
- Two tbsp. (25 grams) diced tomato
- Half avocado, diced

INSTRUCTIONS:

1. Before you start cooking, make sure everything is broken up. In a mixing dish, combine sour cream, paprika, and salt. Now, follow Dana's Easy Omelet Method to make your omelet. When the bottom is done, add the ham and tomato, cover, and reduce the heat to light.

2. Allow for a minute or two for the top to set.

3. To eat, arrange avocado slices on top of the ham and tomato, fold the omelet, and finish with seasoned sour cream.

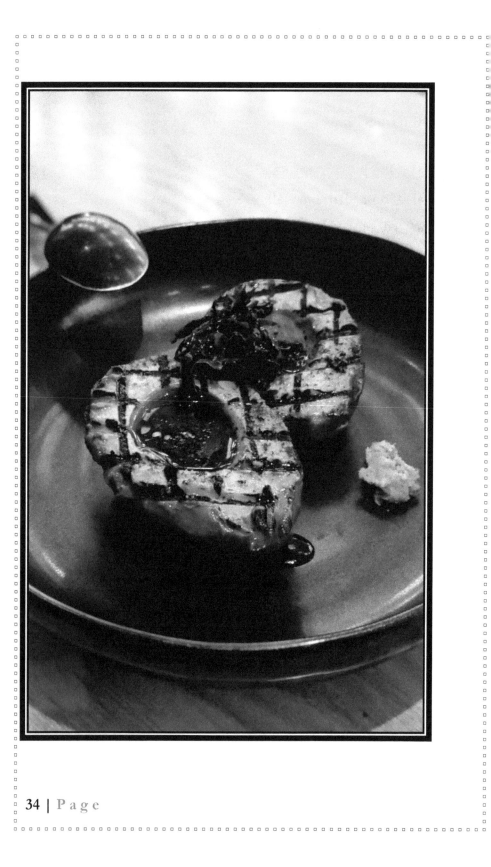

LUNCH

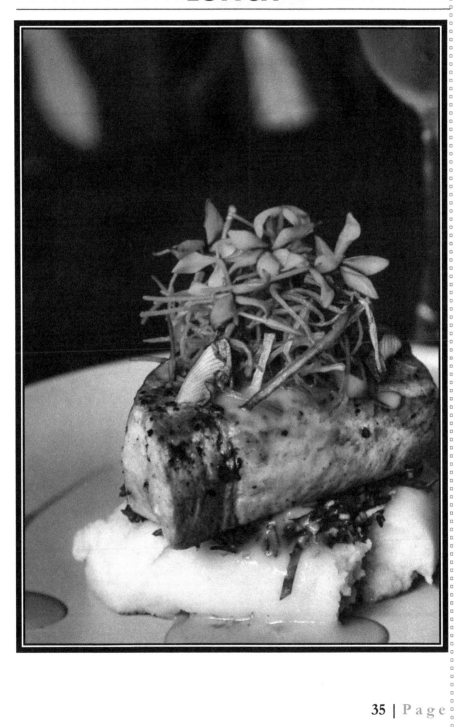

12. ROASTED RED PEPPER SANDWICH

Servings: 4

Cooking Time: 25 Minutes

Calories: 350

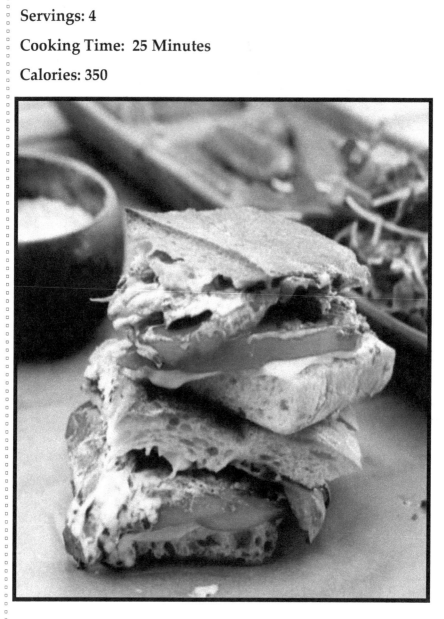

INGREDIENTS:

- One whole-wheat pita loaf
- Two big pieces Roasted Peppers
- 1 oz. hard Parmesan-Reggiano cheddar cheese,
- Four–six Romaine lettuce leaves, broken
- Salt and freshly ground pepper to taste

INSTRUCTIONS:

1. Split the pita loaf in two, open the pockets on either side and gently barbecue. Break Parmesan-Reggiano cheddar cheese, sprouts, and lettuce and place one large piece of roasted pepper in each half pita bag.

2. Season to taste with salt and pepper in each bag. Serve with olives as a garnish.

13. **HEALTHY VEGGIE WRAP**

Servings: 2

Cooking Time: 25 Minutes

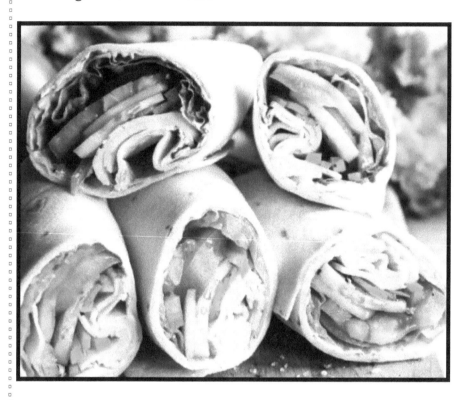

INGREDIENTS:

- Olive oil cooking drizzle
- Third-fourth tbsp. cut down into pieces dried oregano
- One-fourth tbsp. cut down into pieces dried rosemary
- Third-fourth tsp. dried thyme
- Half (15-oz.) can chickpeas, rinsed and drained one-fourth tsp. cumin

- Salt and freshly ground pepper to taste
- Six whole wheat flat bread (eight–ten-inch),
- Warmed Alfalfa sprouts
- Two moderate tomatoes,
- One green bell pepper, cut into strips
- Two moderate zucchinis,

INSTRUCTIONS:

1. Cooking drizzle can be used to coat a nonstick pan. Drizzle olive oil over tomatoes, cucumbers, onions, green bell pepper, and zucchini in a sauce. Roast for 15–20 minutes at 425 degrees with oregano, rosemary, and thyme drizzled on top.

2. Add the chickpeas, cumin, salt, and pepper to taste, and cook for another 15–20 minutes, or until tender. Fill a warmed flatbread with bean and vegetable filling. Top with a mash-up. Fill warmed flat bread with bean and veggie Merge, top with alfalfa sprouts, if need, roll up, and serve.

14. GLUTEN-FREE CRAB AND AVOCADO STUFFED PITA POCKETS

Servings: 4

Cooking Time: 20 Minutes

Calories: 350

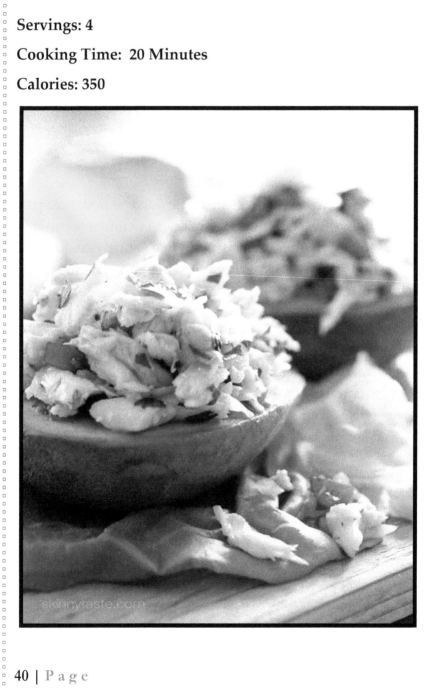

INGREDIENTS:

- Two-third mug light mayonnaise
- Four tbsp. fresh lemon juice
- Three tbsp. finely chopped white onion
- Salt and freshly ground pepper to taste
- Four whole-grain pita loaves, cut in half one mug of alfalfa sprouts
- Two tbsp. chopped Roasted Peppers Pinch cayenne pepper
- One lb. (about two mugs) lump crabmeat,
- Well-drained one mug chopped precooked shrimp
- Two little avocados, chopped

INSTRUCTIONS:

1. Freeze mayonnaise, lemon juice, roasted pepper, and cayenne before ready to use (about one hour). Combine lobster, shrimp, avocados, onion, salt, and pepper to taste in a mixing dish.

2. Fill half of each pita loaf with crab batter and one-eighth of the mayonnaise batter. Fill each pita with a one-eighth mug of alfalfa sprouts and eat.

15. FAT-FREE GRILLED JUMBO PORTOBELLO MUSHROOM SANDWICH

Servings: 3

Cooking Time: 20 Minutes

Calories: 350

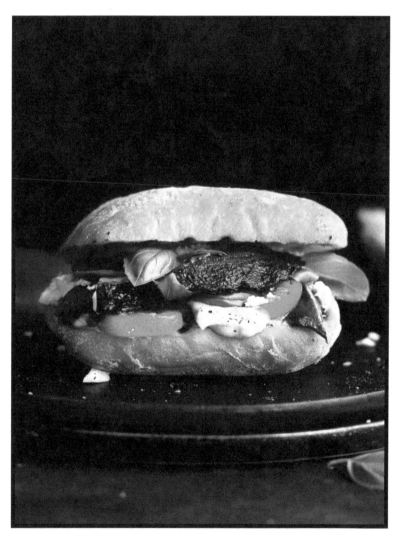

INGREDIENTS:

- Four larges (four–six-inch) portobello mushrooms
- Salt and freshly ground pepper to taste four whole-grain hamburger buns
- Condiments of choice
- One tbsp. Balsamic vinegar
- One tbsp. Worcestershire sauce
- One-third mug Extra-virgin olive oil

INSTRUCTIONS:

1. Wash and clean mushrooms. Merge along with vinegar, Worcestershire sauce, olive oil, salt and pepper, then place mushrooms during a re-sealable plastic baggie and place batter over mushrooms. Seal bag and gently toss mushrooms and marinade to hide mushrooms. Freeze and marinate for one-two hours.

2. Warm-up grill, place mushrooms on the grill, and brush tops with remaining marinade. Grille, each facet for five-half-dozen minutes or until mushrooms a, re soft. Turn mushrooms over once, brushing marinade batter onto alternative side before grilling. Put on a whole-grain bun and add condiments of alternative, if need.

16. FAT-FREE JUMBO WITH MUSHROOMS

Servings: 3

Cooking Time: 20 Minutes

Calories: 350

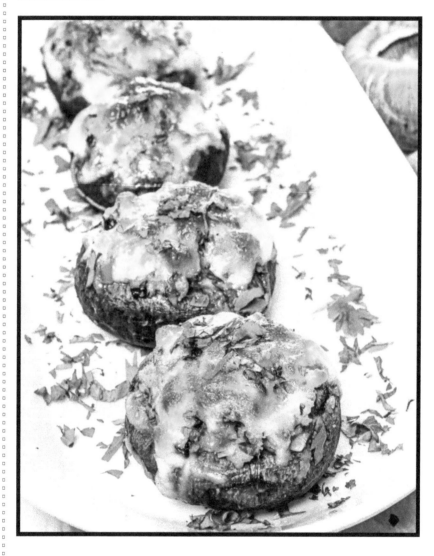

INGREDIENTS:

- Garlic salt to taste
- One-half p. Extra-virgin olive oil
- One-fourth tsp. balsamic glaze
- Half a moderate red onion, finely diced
- Ten moderate pitted black olives
- Four (six-inch) pita loaves
- Two tbsp. stone-ground mustard
- One tsp. Finely chopped fresh cilantro, two cloves fresh garlic, finely crushed
- One-eighth tsp. freshly ground pepper
- One-half mugs shredded lettuce
- Half mug chopped carrot
- Half mug diced celery
- One big tomato, diced
- Four oz. cut down into pieces feta cheddar cheese

INSTRUCTIONS:

1. Divide pita loaves crosswise in half, spread open pockets (to keep from sealing shut), and lightly grill. Roll out a skinny layer of mustard within of toasted pockets.

2. Put aside. Merge cilantro, garlic, pepper, and garlic salt with olive oil and glaze; beat along to blend well and then set aside. Merge onion, olives, lettuce, carrot, celery, and tomato, toss to Merge and fill pockets with the vegetable blend. Drizzle each stuffed loaf with glaze batter and add bog down into items feta cheddar cheese. Serve right away.

17. Spicy Hummus in Toasted Pita Loaves

Servings: 1

Cooking Time: 20 Minutes

Calories: 350

Ingredients:

- One big clove fresh garlic
- Two tbsp. tahini paste
- One (15-oz.) can chickpeas, well rinsed and drained Juice from one lemon
- One-fourth mug water
- Dash of salt

Instructions:

1. Add a pinch of red-hot pepper flakes, crushed three whole wheat pita loaves (six inches), eight tomato slices, peeled and finely sliced half cucumber (one-fourth inch thick) Sprouts of alfalfa Blend chickpeas, lemon juice, and water in a food processor until desired consistency is achieved. Blend in the garlic, tahini paste, cinnamon, and warm pepper flakes.

2. Cut pita loaves in half and grill lightly. Divide batter into four portions and stuff loaves with batter. Wrap every half loaf with tomato, cucumber, and alfalfa sprouts.

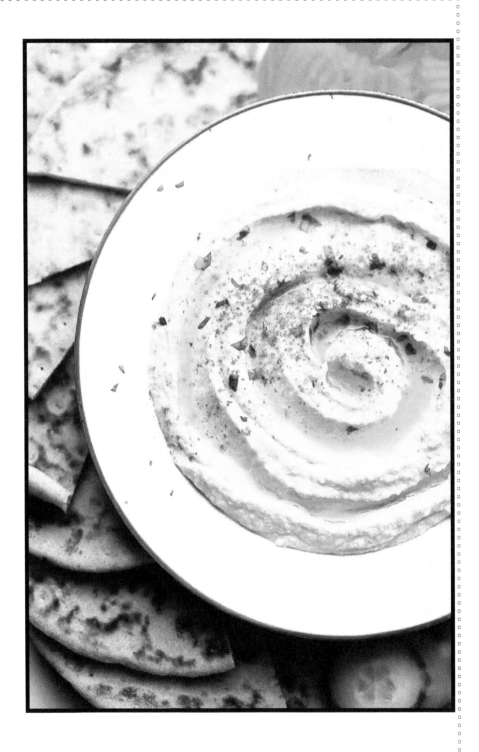

18. Hummus in Grilled Pita Loaves

Servings: 3

Cooking Time: 20 Minutes

Calories: 350

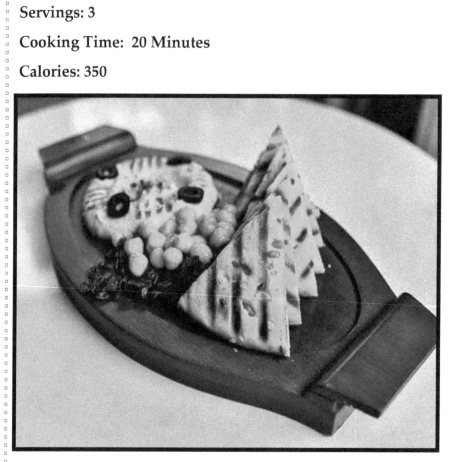

Ingredients:

- One-third mug thinly diced celery
- Half moderate cucumber, diced
- One-fourth mug finely chopped onion

- One-fourth mug light mayonnaise

- One tbsp. balsamic nectar

- One (15-oz.) can chickpeas, rinsed and drained

- One mug of shredded fresh spinach

- Two-third mug halved seedless red grapes

- Half mug finely chopped red bell pepper

- Half tbsp. poppy seeds

- Four (six-inch) whole wheat pita loaves, cut in half

INSTRUCTIONS:

1. Merge chickpeas, spinach, grapes, red bell pepper, celery, cucumber, and onion. Beat together mayonnaise, balsamic nectar, and poppy seeds.

2. Put poppy seed batter to chickpea batter and beat until well blended. Lightly grill pita halves and fill with chickpea filling. Serve right away.

19. CHICKPEA AND FRESH SPINACH SANDWICH

Servings: 3

Cooking Time: 20 Minutes

Calories: 350

INGREDIENTS:

- Salt and freshly ground pepper to taste
- One (15-oz.) can chickpeas
- Two tsp. Extra-virgin olive oil
- Two cloves fresh garlic, minced
- Half moderate white onion, diced
- One clove of fresh garlic, cut in half
- Five–six oz. fresh spinach leaves

INSTRUCTIONS:

1. Chickpeas should be properly rinsed and drained. Set aside after mashing to a paste. Fry garlic and onion in one tsp olive oil until golden brown. Place chickpea paste, salt, pepper to taste, and warm pepper flakes, if desired, in a mixing dish.

2. Place aside the remaining tsp. of olive oil to drizzle over the pastes. Toast whole wheat bread slices and rub fresh garlic halves on one side of each piece. Divide paste batter and spinach leaves into four portions and make into four sandwiches. Serve.

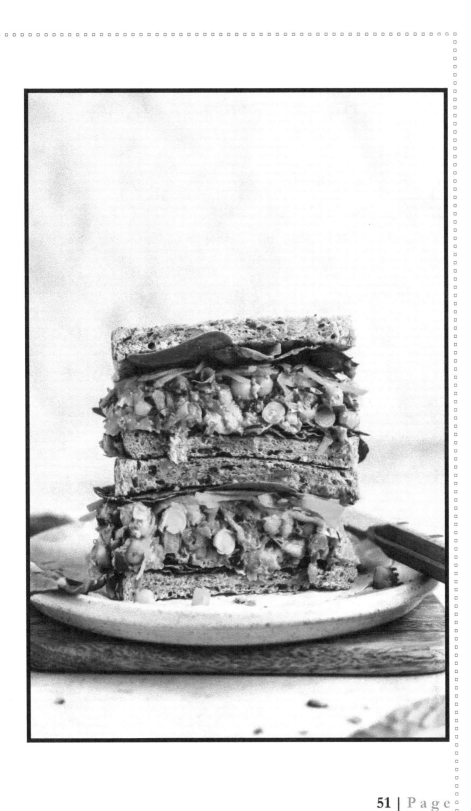

20. AMAZING SMOKED FISH AND ROASTED PEPPER SANDWICH

Servings: 1

Cooking Time: 20 Minutes

Calories: 350

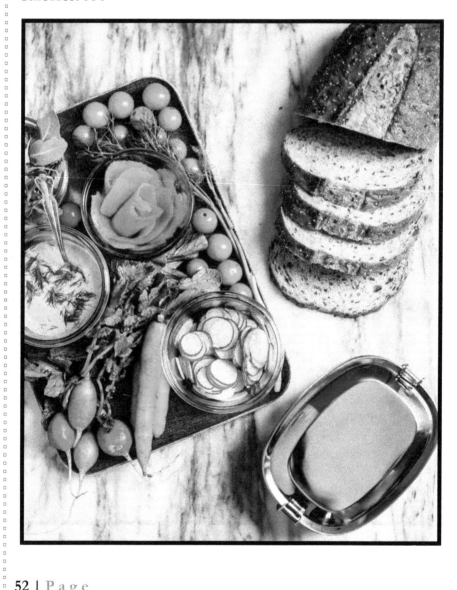

INGREDIENTS:

- Two tbsp. Extra-virgin olive oil
- One clove fresh garlic, mashed into a paste eight slices whole wheat grain bread
- Three oz. Smoked fish
- Four tbsp. Shredded romaine lettuce four tsp. Diced toasted Peppers
- Two tsp. light mayonnaise

INSTRUCTIONS:

1. One tsp. Olive oil is set aside after combining olive oil and garlic.

2. Brush all sides of the bread with the batter and grill for four minutes at 350 degrees, until golden brown. Remove from the equation.

3. Combine the tuna, basil, and roasted peppers in a mixing dish; set aside.

4. Combine mayonnaise and reserved olive oil in a mixing dish and stir into the fish batter.

5. Prepare four sandwiches by dividing the batter into four servings and spreading it on toast.

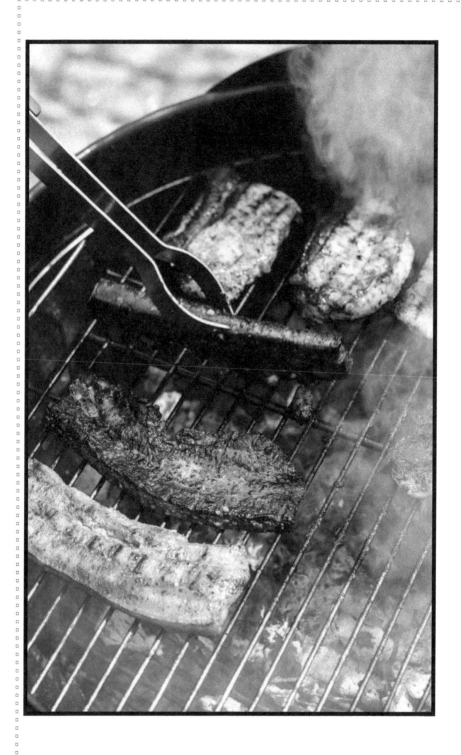

DINNER

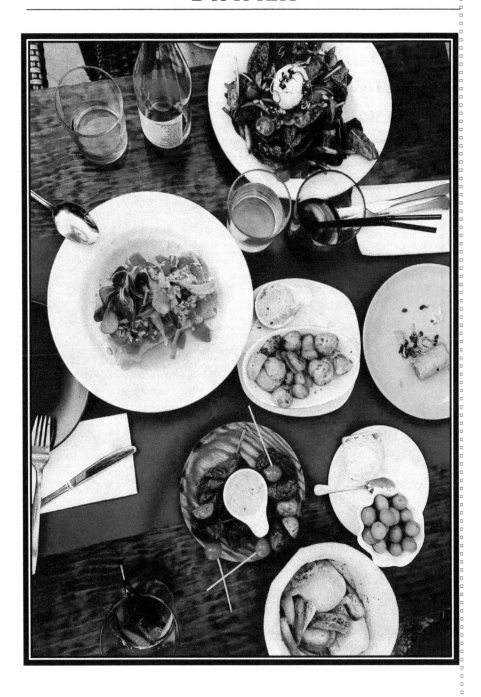

21. AMAZING SHRIMP AND AVOCADO WRAP

Servings: 2

Cooking Time: 20 Minutes

Calories: 300

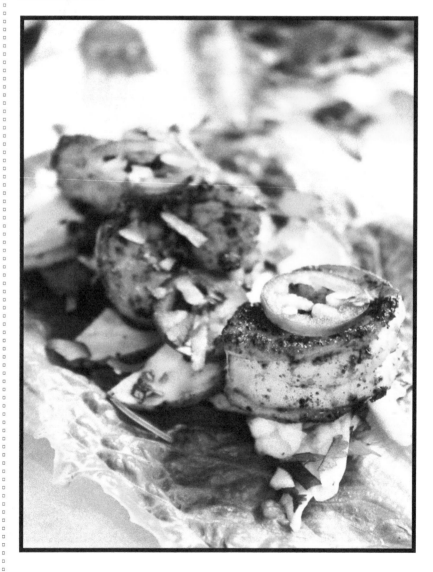

INGREDIENTS:

- Half clove fresh garlic, finely minced
- Two tbsp. Finely chopped red onion half tsp. freshly squeezed lime
- Juice Salt and freshly ground pepper to taste
- Two (ten-inch) whole grain wraps
- Two tbsp. prepared basil pesto
- Half ripened avocado, pitted, peeled, and diced into eight wedges
- One mug baby spinach leaves, divided
- Ten big cooked shrimp, deveined and peeled, divided

INSTRUCTIONS:

1. Put wraps on a clean, flat surface and unfold one tbsp of pesto over prime of each wrap. Organize four wedges of avocado down the center of every wrap. Drizzle garlic and onion over avocado.

2. Drizzle on a little amount of lime juice. Season with salt and pepper. Divide spinach and shrimp into two parts, adding a bed of spinach to every wrap, followed by shrimp on prime.

3. Fold over the high and bottom of every wrap and, starting at one finish, tightly roll up the wrap. Secure with big tooth decide if necessary. Cut wrap in half on diagonal and serve.

22. Ginger-and Sesame-Infused Carrot and Cucumber Salad

Servings: 3

Cooking Time: 20 Minutes

Calories: 300

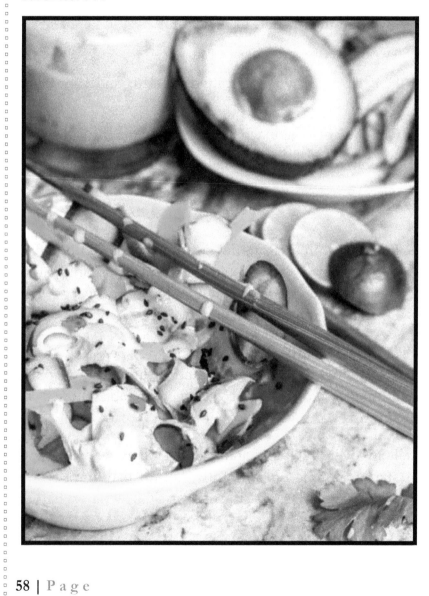

INGREDIENTS:

- Two tsp. tamarind paste
- Two tbsp. (30 milliliters) rice vinegar
- Two tbsp. (30 milliliters) water
- Two tsp. to Toasted sesame oil
- Two tsp. Grated ginger root
- Two cloves' garlic, grated
- Two big-size carrots, peeled and shredded
- One English cucumber, cut in half lengthwise and finely diced into half-moons
- One-half tsp. Poppy seeds
- One-half tsp. sesame seeds
- Two tbsp. (12 grams) finely chopped scallion
- Half tsp. fine sea salt, to taste

INSTRUCTIONS:

1. Heat the oil in a large frying pan over medium heat, then add the ginger and garlic and cook until fragrant. Mix the tamarind paste, vinegar, and water until the tamarind is fully dissolved. Place the shredded carrots in a dish and set them aside for a few minutes. Toss the cucumber half-moons with the carrots and sauce in a large mixing tub. Drizzle the poppy seeds, sesame seeds, scallions (if need), and salt on top. Chill for one hour and beat before serving.

23. CRANBERRY CHILI

Servings: 3

Cooking Time: 20 Minutes

Calories: 300

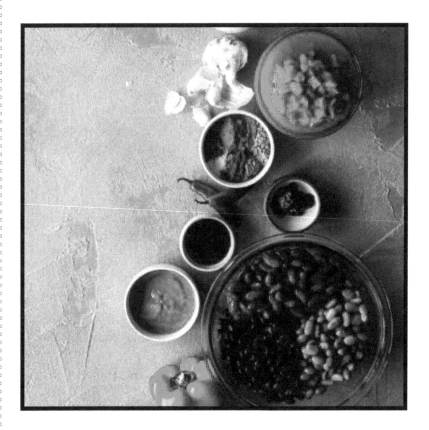

INGREDIENTS:

- Two tbsp. (30 milliliters) tequila

- Half tsp. coarse sea salt

- Six oz. (170 grams) fresh or frozen cranberries

- One can (15 oz., or 425 grams) diced tomatoes with jalapeño, including liquid
- Half mug (120 milliliters) water
- One tbsp. (15 milliliters) Extra-virgin olive oil
- One mug (213 grams) diced red onion
- Two tbsp. (16 grams) mild to moderate chili powder
- One-fourth tsp. Cayenne pepper, to taste
- One tsp. ground cumin
- One tbsp. (21 grams) agave nectar
- One can (15 oz., or 425 grams) cooked red kidney beans, drained and rinsed

INSTRUCTIONS:

1. In a huge-size pan, the temperature of the oil over moderate-hot temperature. Put the chopped onion and prepare till tender, for four minutes, moving often.

2. Beat within the chili powder, cayenne, and cumin. Prepare for one minute, until fragrant. Put the agave, tequila, and salt, moving well.

3. Beat within the cranberries and let prepare for five minutes. Put the tomatoes, their liquid, and the water. Carry to a low boil, cover with a lid, and reduce the temperature to a stew. Let stew for 15 minutes. Beat in the beans, cowl again, and let stew for another 15 minutes. If the chili is simply too liquid for you, let it quiet down for another number of minutes, uncovered.

24. BARLEY CHILI

Servings: 4

Cooking Time: 20 Minutes

Calories: 300

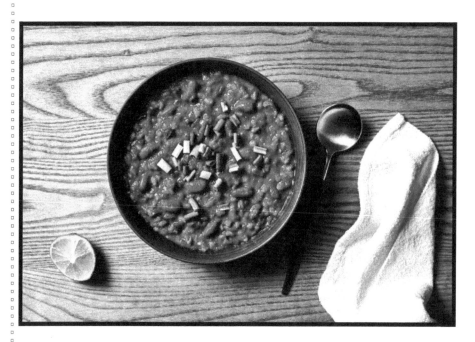

INGREDIENTS:

- Half tsp. coarse sea salt, to taste
- Two tbsp. (16 grams) mild to moderate chili powder
- One tbsp. (six grams) ground cumin
- One-fourth tsp. Cayenne pepper, to taste
- Two tsp. dried oregano

- One mug (200 grams) uncooked pearl barley, rinsed and drained
- One tbsp. (15 milliliters) Extra-virgin olive oil
- One big-size carrot, finely diced
- One big-size zucchini, finely diced
- One mug (160 grams) chopped onion
- Two big-size cloves garlic, grated
- Three mugs (705 milliliters) water or vegetable broth
- Two tbsp. (33 grams) tomato paste
- One can (15 oz., or 425 grams) tomato sauce
- One can (15 oz., or 425 grams) cooked black beans, drained and rinsed

INSTRUCTIONS:

1. In a big-size pan, the oil's temperature over moderate-high temperature and add the carrot, zucchini, onion, garlic, and salt. Prepare for five minutes over moderate temperature. Put the chili powder, cumin, cayenne, and oregano, and prepare for one minute until fragrant. Put the barley, and prepare for an additional two minutes.

2. Put the water, tomato paste, and tomato sauce. Beat well. Carry to a boil, cover with a lid, and let stew for thirty-five minutes, moving every current and then making certain the barley does not follow the pan. Take out the lid, beat in the beans, and let the remaining liquid cut back over low temperature, with the dish uncovered, for another ten minutes, or until the barley is tender. Therefore, the chili is at you would like consistency.

25. CHINESE CHICKEN NOODLE SOUP

Servings: 3

Cooking Time: 20 Minutes

Calories: 300

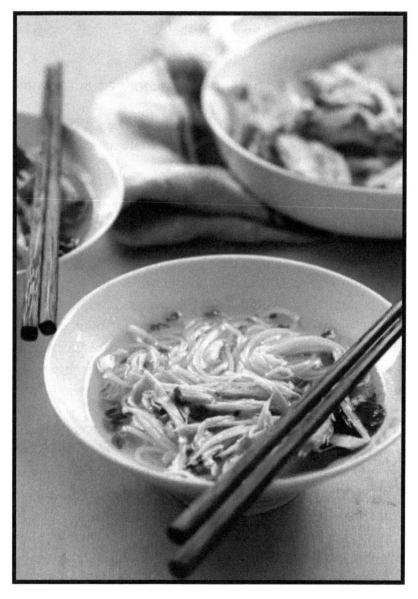

INGREDIENTS:

- One mug (135 grams)of fresh, frozen, or canned corn
- Six oz. (170 grams) dry upon, soba
- Four mugs (940 milliliters,) chicken-flavored vegetable broth, or more if you want a
- More brothy soup
- One mug (135 grams) of fresh, frozen, or canned peas

INSTRUCTIONS:

1. Carry the broth to a boil in a moderate-size dish.

2. Put the peas, corn, and tofu, and return to a boil.

3. Put the noodles and stew for seven to 15 minutes, or until the noodles are tender.

26. Coconut Curry Carrot Soup

Servings: 1

Cooking Time: 20 Minutes

Calories: 300

Ingredients:

- One tbsp. (six grams) yellow curry powder, store-bought or homemade
- One tbsp. (15 grams) minced garlic
- Salt and pepper, to taste
- Two mugs (470 milliliters) vegetable broth
- One can (14 oz., or 414 milliliters) coconut milk
- One lb. (455 grams) peeled carrots

Instructions:

1. Put all the ingredients into a dish and carry them to a boil.
2. Decrease to a stew and stew until the carrots are nice and tender, about 15 minutes.
3. Using an immersion or a countertop blender, stir until glossy.

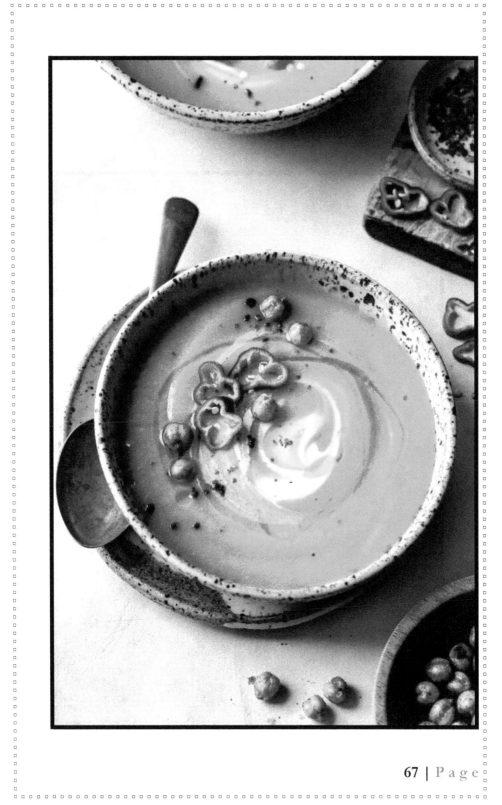

27. **RUSTIC POTATO LEEK SOUP**

Servings: 2

Cooking Time: 20 Minutes

Calories: 300

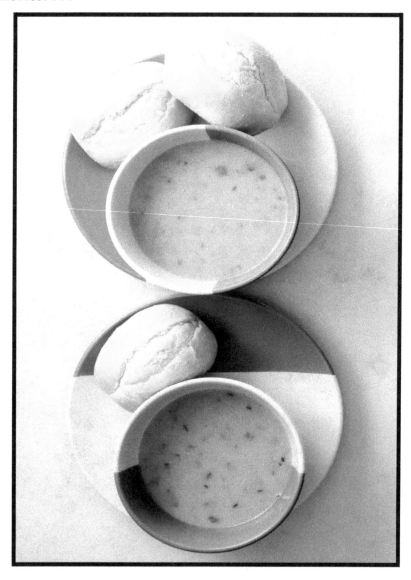

INGREDIENTS:

- Two tbsp. (eight grams) finely chopped lemongrass
- Four mugs (940 milliliters,) vegetable broth
- Two leeks
- Two tbsp. (28 grams) nondairy butter
- One half lb. (690 grams) russet potatoes
- Salt and pepper, to taste

INSTRUCTIONS:

1. Cut the leeks into one-fourth-in. (six-mm) slices, using most of the leek, up till it forks off into separate leaves.

2. Put the butter into a dish and melt over hot temperature. Put the leeks and lemongrass and fry till baked, concerning two minutes.

3. Put the broth, deglaze the pan, and carry it to a boil.

4. Put the potatoes, reduce to a stew, cowl, and stew for thirty minutes.

5. Using an immersion or a countertop blender, blend until swish but still a small amount chunky. Season with salt and pepper.

28. RATATOUILLE WITH WHITE BEANS

Servings: 2

Cooking Time: 20 Minutes

Calories: 300

INGREDIENTS:

- One little zucchini, chopped
- Two moderate tomatoes, chopped
- One tsp. every of dried parsley, thyme, and
- Rosemary; if fresh, one tbsp. of every
- One-fourth Cup olive oil
- Two baby eggplants, chopped
- One onion, diced
- Two cloves' garlic, minced
- Salt and pepper to taste
- One (13-oz.) can of white beans

INSTRUCTIONS:

1. Warm up the olive oil. Fry the eggplant, onion, garlic, and zucchini for five minutes. Put tomatoes, herbs, salt, and pepper. Wrap and stew for 15 minutes. Warm the beans and serve by pouring vegetables over the beans.

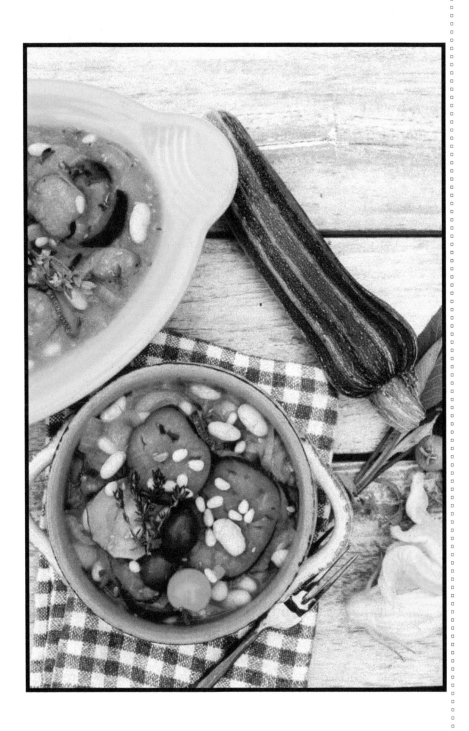

29. COCONUT CREAM OF MUSHROOM SOUP

Servings: 1

Cooking Time: 20 Minutes

Calories: 300

INGREDIENTS:

- Two tbsp. (30 grams) minced garlic
- Two cans (14 oz., or 414 milliliters every) coconut milk
- Salt and pepper, to taste
- Two tbsp. (28 grams) nondairy butter
- Eight oz. (227 grams) button mushrooms, diced
- Eight oz. (227 grams) portobello mushroom caps, diced
- Shredded coconut for garnish

INSTRUCTIONS:

1. Melt the butter in a pan and fry the mushrooms and garlic for seven to 15 minutes, or until the mushrooms have shrunk in size by about half.

2. Put the coconut milk and carry it to a boil. Decrease to a stew and stew for 15 minutes. Using an immersion or a countertop blender, stir until glossy. Season with salt and pepper and garnish with the shredded coconut.

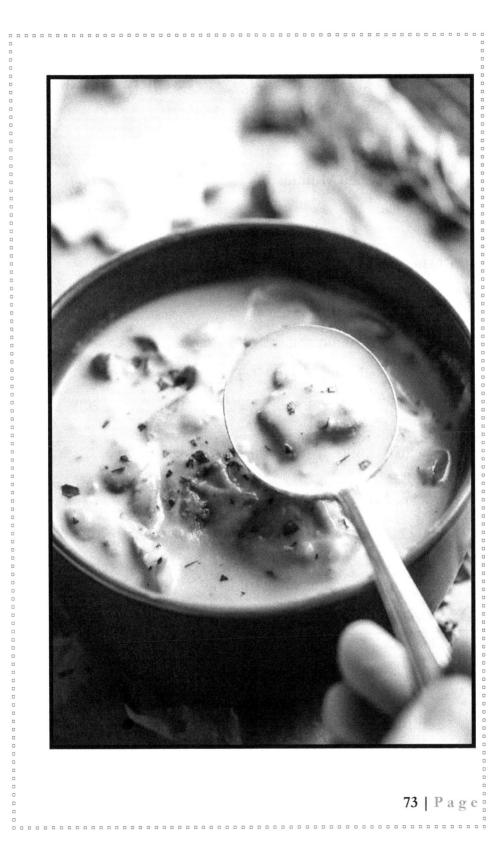

30. GLUTEN-FREE SOUTHWESTERN BEAN AND CORN SOUP

Servings: 2

Cooking Time: 20 Minutes

Calories: 300

INGREDIENTS:

- Half tsp. Ground cumin
- One tsp. Ground chipotles powder
- One tsp. ground coriander
- One half mugs (375 grams) fresh, frozen, or canned corn
- One half mugs (390 grams) fully cooked pinto or black beans
- Two tbsp. (28 grams) nondairy butter
- One big-size red onion, roughly chopped or diced Pinch salt
- Two tbsp. (30 grams) minced garlic
- One mug (235 milliliters) vegetable broth
- One mug (227 grams) tomato sauce
- Diced scallion, plus more for garnish
- Nondairy sour cream, store-bought or homemade for garnish

INSTRUCTIONS:

1. Melt the butter during a dish over-warm temperature.

2. Put the onion and a pinch of salt, and fry till caramelized, for 15 minutes, usually moving to stop burning.

3. Put the garlic, and fry a pair of to three minutes a lot.

4. Put the broth, and deglaze the dish.

5. Put the tomato sauce, cumin, chipotle, and coriander.

6. Carry to a boil, then reduce to a stew.

7. Put the corn and beans and stew for ten to 15 minutes. Beat within the soymilk, if using, and come to a boil.

8. Take out from the temperature and beat within the one mug scallions.

9. Serve garnished with further scallions and nondairy sour cream.

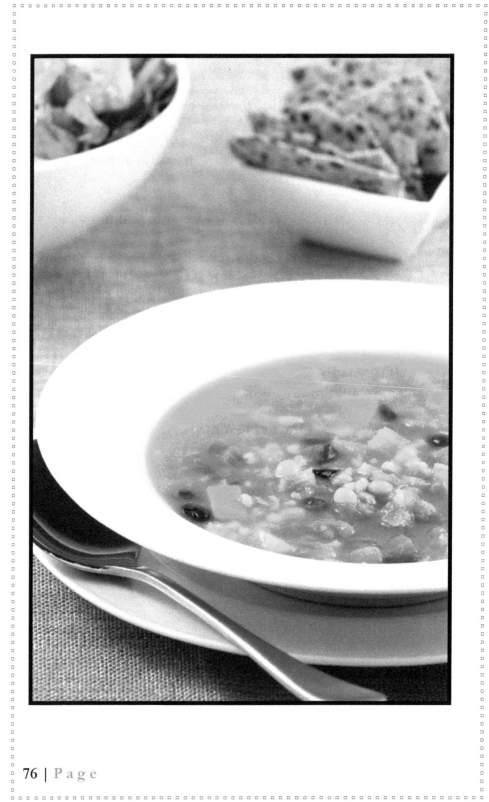

SNACKS

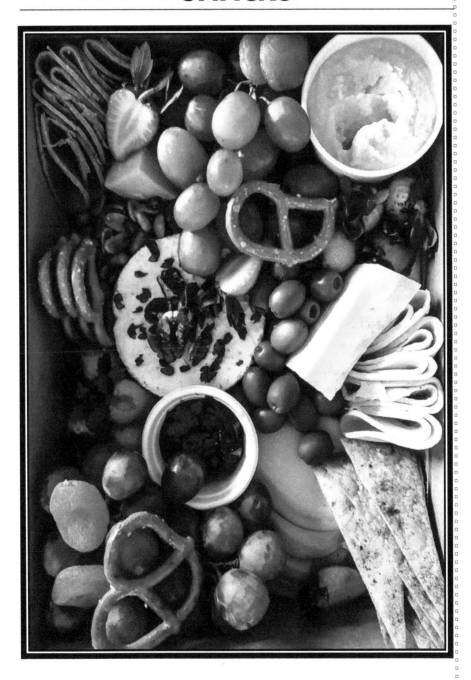

31. ITALIAN CROSTINI

Servings: 2

Cooking Time: 15 Minutes

Calories: 150

INGREDIENTS:

- Extra-virgin olive oil cooking drizzle
- Two half tsp. fresh garlic paste
- One French baguette roughly ten–12 inches long,
- Minced dry or fresh basil, parsley, or chives
- Salt and freshly ground pepper to Taste

INSTRUCTIONS:

1. Drizzle a small amount of cooking oil on both sides of each slice of bread. Apply a small number of garlic paste to one side of each slice, then drizzle the herb of choice over the garlic. Season to taste with salt and pepper.

2. Place slices on a nonstick baking sheet and bake until light golden brown (about three-five minutes) in a 375°F oven on the middle rack.

3. Serve as is or add your favorite topping (smoked mozzarella, chopped fresh tomatoes, chopped black olives, roasted garlic, etc.) if need.

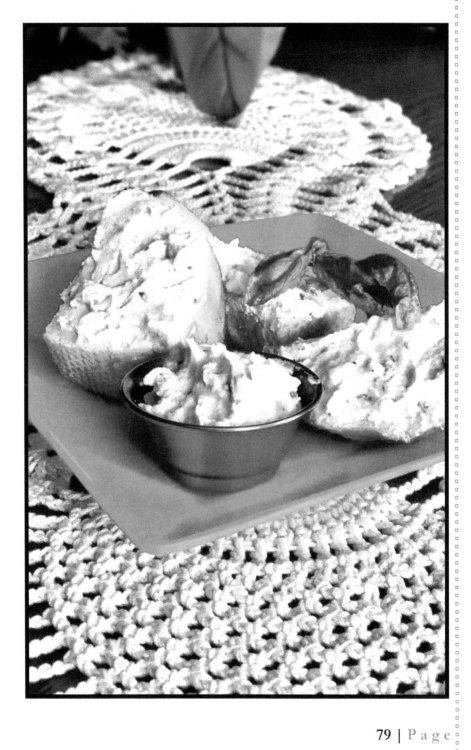

32. BABY SHRIMP ON TOASTED RYE

Servings: 3

Cooking Time: 15 Minutes

Calories: 150

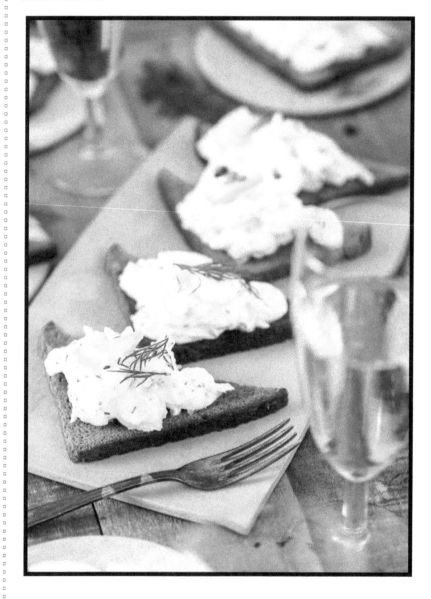

INGREDIENTS:

- Half tsp. chopped capers
- 16 slices cocktail-sized, thin rye bread Garlic/olive oil cooking drizzle
- One bag cooked salad shrimp, thawed
- Half mug reduced-fat mayonnaise
- Two tbsp. Finely minced shallot
- One tbsp. Finely chopped fresh parsley one tsp. Dijon mustard
- Scant splash of freshly squeezed lemon juice 16 paper-thin slices lemon

INSTRUCTIONS:

1. Combine mayonnaise, shallot, parsley, mustard, and capers in a little dish. Wrap in plastic wrap and chill for at least one hour to mix flavors.

2. Meanwhile, softly drizzle rye slices with garlic/olive oil drizzle and barbecue until mildly crispy in a toaster oven or oven at 300 degrees.

3. Remove the rye grill from the oven and sprinkle one teaspoon of the mayonnaise batter on each sandwich. Wrap with four-five shrimp and a little splash of lemon juice. Put a slice of lemon for garnish and serve.

33. APPLE, GORGONZOLA, AND WALNUT

Servings: 1

Cooking Time: 15 Minutes

Calories: 150

INGREDIENTS:

- Two Granny Smith apples, cored and thinly diced
- Eight oz. cut down into pieces
- 24 thin slices of French bread
- Olive oil cooking drizzle
- Gorgonzola cheddar cheese
- One mug of chopped walnuts

INSTRUCTIONS:

1. Preheat the broiler. Drizzle a small amount of cooking oil on both sides of the bread slices. Place slices on a baking sheet and broil until lightly browned on both sides, rotating once. Remove the broiler from the oven and put two apple slices on each piece of barbecue.

2. Wrap a mound of gorgonzola cheddar cheese around each piece. Press walnut pieces into cheddar cheese and return to broiler. Grill until cheddar cheese melts and both cheddar cheese and walnuts are lightly baked. Serve while warm.

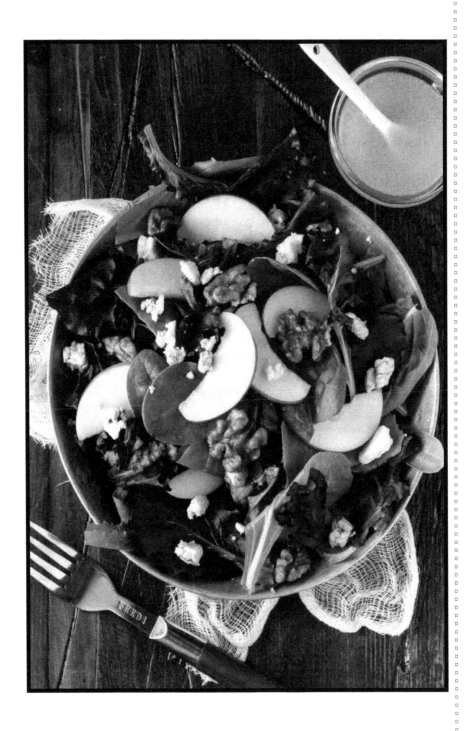

34. Avocado and Mango Salsa

Servings: 1

Cooking Time: 15 Minutes

Calories: 150

INGREDIENTS:

- Half red onion, finely chopped
- One ripened avocado, peeled
- Two ripened mangoes, peeled and
- Cut into half-inch cubes half jalapeño pepper,
- Two tbsp. fresh cilantro, finely chopped Juice from one lime
- Salt and freshly ground pepper to taste

INSTRUCTIONS:

1. Merge onion, avocado, mango, jalapeño, cilantro, and lime juice in a dish.
2. Blend well to incorporate ingredients. Season with salt and pepper to taste. Wrap and refrigerate to chill. Use as topping for fish or as a dip with chips.

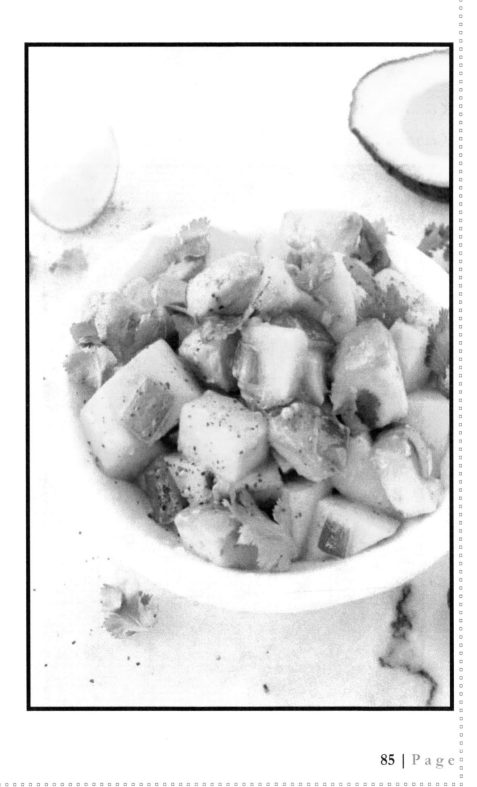

35. DELICIOUS CHEESY CRAB BITES

Servings: 3

Cooking Time: 15 Minutes

Calories: 150

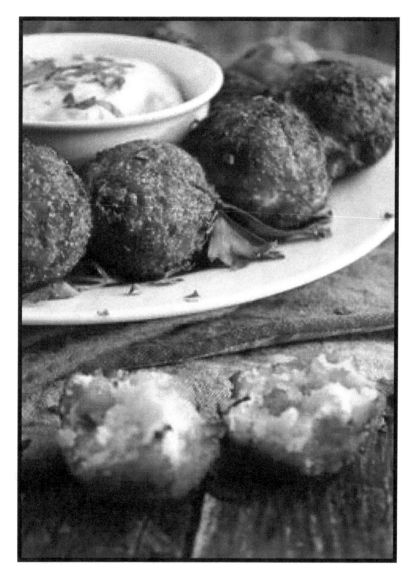

INGREDIENTS:

- Four oz. Low-fat cream cheddar cheese, softened
- One-fourth mug low-fat shredded cheddar
- One tsp. Freshly squeezed lemon juice
- Half tsp. Seafood seasoning Merge
- Half tsp. garlic powder
- One scallion, thinly diced
- Dash of paprika

INSTRUCTIONS:

1. Preheat the oven to 350 degrees Fahrenheit.

2. Cream together cream cheddar cheese, cheddar cheese, mayonnaise, and lemon juice in a mixing dish.

3. Mix in the fish seasoning, garlic powder, scallions, and crabmeat.

4. Fill phyllo shells halfway with the batter, cover with a splash of paprika, and put on a flat baking sheet.

5. Oven for roughly 15 minutes, or until shells are golden brown and the batter is heated through.

6. Serve warm.

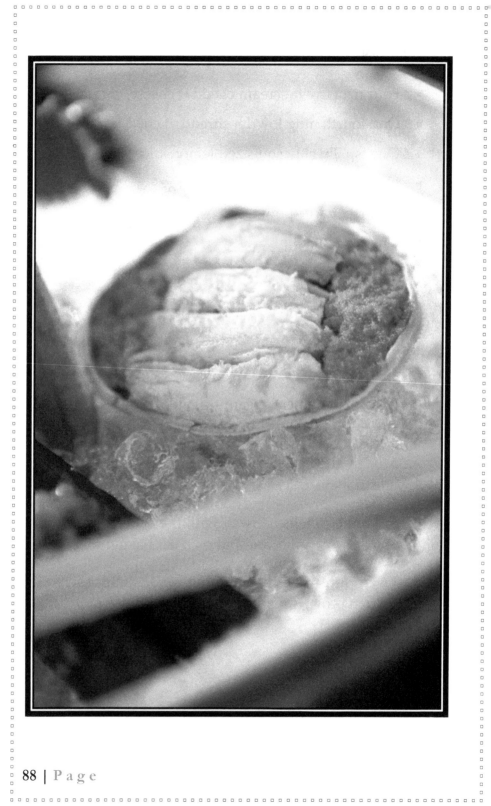

DESSERTS

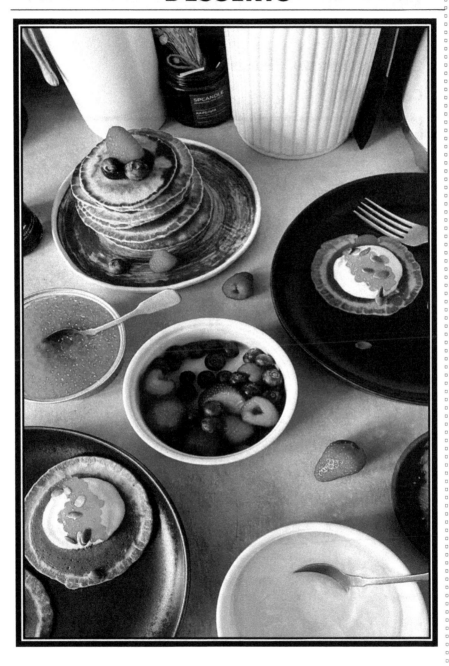

36. Crème De Banana Baked Apples

Servings: 2

Cooking Time: 20 Minutes

Calories: 300

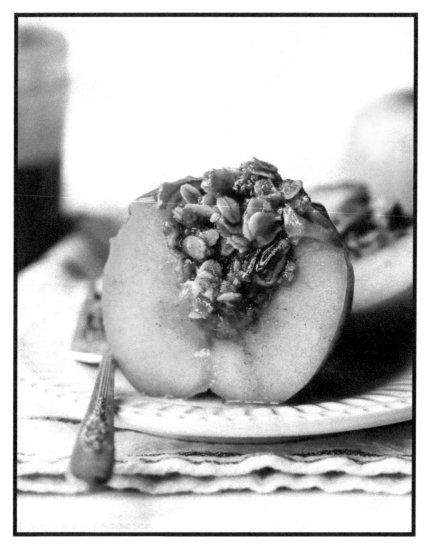

INGREDIENTS:

- Four moderate sweet apples, peeled, cored, and
- Halved six oz. Unsweetened apple juice
- Two tsp. Ground cinnamon
- Three tbsp. Pure honey
- One tsp. Vanilla essence
- Four tbsp. Crème de Banana liqueur
- One mug plain fat-free yogurt
- Non-caloric sweetener to taste

INSTRUCTIONS:

1. Put apples cored facet up in a very snugly fitting shallow baking dish. Put apple juice to only barely cowl bottom halves of apples. Drizzle with one tsp. Cinnamon, cowl, and oven for 30-40 minutes during a 350degree oven or till apples are virtually tender.

2. Take out from the oven and place off any additional liquid, leaving simply enough to cover the bottom of the dish. Merge along with honey, vanilla essence, and liqueur and drizzle over the tops of apples.

3. Drizzle remaining tsp. of cinnamon over prime. Oven for a further ten minutes. Take out from the oven and divide equally onto four dessert plates. Blend yogurt and sweetener and serve on the side.

37. LOW CARB STRAWBERRIES AND BALSAMIC SYRUP

Servings: 2

Cooking Time:

20 Minutes

Calories: 300

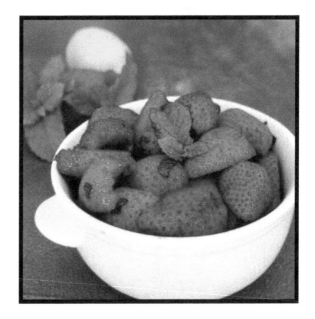

INGREDIENTS:

- Two half mugs fresh strawberries, hulled and halved four tbsp. Crème de
- Banana liqueur
- Non-caloric sweetener to taste
- Balsamic nectar

INSTRUCTIONS:

1. Merge strawberries and liqueur in a big dish, toss well, cover, and refrigerate for 20–30 minutes. When ready to serve, take out strawberries with a slotted spoon and place them in a single layer on a dessert platter.

2. Dust generously with sweetener, drizzle with balsamic nectar and serve.

38. PUMPKIN PUDDING

Servings: 3

Cooking Time: 20 Minutes

Calories: 300

INGREDIENTS:

- Third-fourth mugs skim milk
- One (one-oz.) package sugar-free instant vanilla pudding
- Half mug canned pumpkin
- Half tsp. pumpkin spice

INSTRUCTIONS:

1. Merge cold milk and pudding Merge in a chilled dish and beat until glossy.

2. Blend in pumpkin and spice and refrigerate to chill before serving.

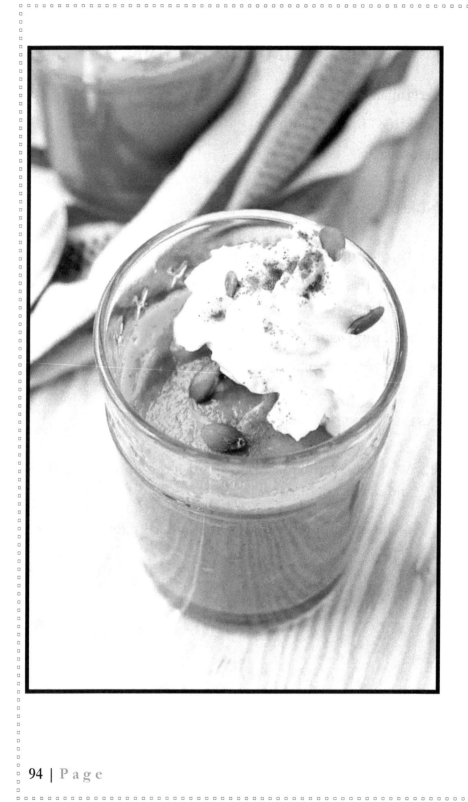

39. STRAWBERRY-RHUBARB QUINOA PUDDING

Servings: 3

Cooking Time: 25 Minutes

Calories: 300

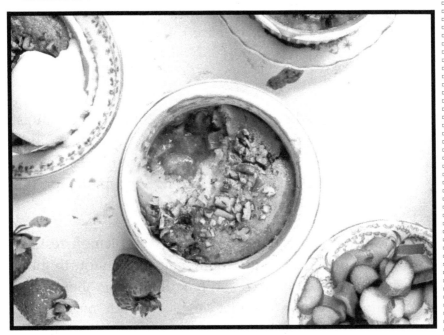

INGREDIENTS:

- Three mugs water, divided
- On one-half chopped rhubarb, fresh or frozen
- One mug chopped strawberries, fresh or frozen, + more for garnish
- Half mug quinoa
- Half tsp. ground cinnamon

- Dash of salt
- One-fourth mug +one-half tsp. Low-calorie baking sweetener half tsp. freshly
- Grated lemon zest
- One tbsp. cornstarch
- One mug plain non-fat yogurt
- One tsp. pure vanilla essence

INSTRUCTIONS:

1. In an exceedingly pan, merge 2third-fourth mugs water, rhubarb, strawberries, quinoa, cinnamon, and salt. Carry to a boil and reduce temperature to a stew. Wrap and prepare for regarding 25 minutes or till quinoa are tender.

2. Beat in one-fourth mug sweetener and lemon zest. A very little dish merges the remaining one-fourth mug water with cornstarch and mix until shiny, then boost quinoa batter and still let stew, constantly moving for one minute. Take out from temperature, divide among vi serving bowls, and refrigerate to cool down for one hour.

3. Meanwhile, merge yogurt, vanilla essence, and the remaining one-half tsp. The sweetener in a very little dish. Wrap each serving with a generous dollop of yogurt batter and diced fresh strawberries.

40. Fat-Free Sweet Mango Mousse

Servings: 3

Cooking Time: 25 Minutes

Calories: 300

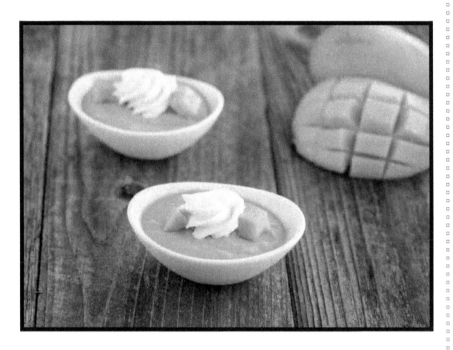

Ingredients:

- Third-fourth mug fresh orange juice
- Two tbsp. orange-flavored liqueur
- One big ripened mango
- One mug of light whipping cream, well chilled
- One-fourth tsp. vanilla essence
- One one-fourth mug water

- One mug couscous

- Four tbsp. Non-caloric sweetener

- One (eight-oz.) container low-fat vanilla yogurt Orange zest

INSTRUCTIONS:

1. Carry water to a boil over moderate-warm temperature. Place couscous slowly, moving once, and remove from temperature. Wrap and put aside for 12-15 minutes till couscous is tender. Put two tbsp. Of sweetener and Merge well into couscous. Wrap and set aside in a little pan over moderate temperature, temperature juice, constantly moving till reduced to the consistency of honey (about four-five minutes).

2. Beat in liqueur. Put aside. Peel the mango; cut half of the flesh into skinny wedges; coarsely dice the opposite half and set aside.

3. Place cream into a calming dish and whip until it peaks. Fold in vanilla essence and remaining sweetener. Divide in half and set half aside. In a clean dish, merge the remaining half of whipped cream, yogurt, and diced mango and refrigerate until well chilled. Before serving, merge mango batter with couscous.

4. Divide into six equal parts, and prime each portion with a smart dollop of the remaining whipped cream and mango wedges. Drizzle with liqueur sauce, drizzle with orange zest and serve.

CONCLUSION

Most diet programs, especially fad detoxes and cleanses, are designed to help people lose weight. However, not everyone on a diet is attempting to shed pounds. Diets can have a variety of outcomes. If you want to enhance your brain health and avoid Alzheimer's disease, you should follow the Brain Health Diet, which has been related to a reduced rate of cognitive decline.

The Brain Health Diet, according to researchers, contains nutrients that may help reduce the creation of beta-amyloid plaques, a possible cause of Alzheimer's disease.

Alzheimer's disease and dementia affect everyone at some point in their lives. Some people are at a higher risk if they have a family history, are over sixty-five, have an unhealthy diet, get little exercise, have high cholesterol, or smoke.

Although there is no research relating the Brain Health Diet to Alzheimer's reversal, there is enough of data to suggest the link between this dietary strategy and Alzheimer's prevention.

It's never too early to start making positive health improvements. Following the Brain Health Diet is the first step in not just lowering your risk but also supplying your body and brain with nutritious foods. The first step in making the shift is to include fresh vegetables, fruits, nuts, olive oil, fish, and chicken in your weekly meals.

The Brain Health Diet combines the DASH and Mediterranean diets to produce a diet that aims to lower the risk of dementia and the deterioration in brain function that many individuals suffer as they become older.

It promotes the eating of a wide variety of vegetables, berries, nuts, olive oil, whole grains, fish, beans, chicken, and wine in moderation. Because butter and margarine, cheese, red meat, fried food, pastries, and sweets are high in saturated and trans-fat, this type of diet recommends minimizing your intake of these foods.

Make sure you start exercising consistently in addition to consuming nutritious foods.

Begin with an easy ten-minute stroll around the neighborhood. You may do a combination of cardio and lifting to maintain your weight while also improving the health of your brain.

Social connections with your pals should be part of your lifestyle.

We are all social animals, and one of the best ways to keep our brains happy and healthy is to engage in positive social interactions.

Apart from that, try to learn something new every day. Maintain a healthy diet, get enough sleep, manage your stress, exercise, socialize, maintain your vascular health, and mentally stimulate yourself.

I hope you learned numerous vital things that will help you keep your brain in excellent condition and condition. We are everyone at danger of acquiring it, but if you follow the seven pillars and eat a healthy Brain Health Diet, you will notice a substantial difference.

Finally, I'd want to express my gratitude for taking the time to read. Maintain a healthy diet, stay active and sociable, lower your stress levels, and keep yourself occupied by doing what you enjoy while surrounded by people who love you and make you happy.

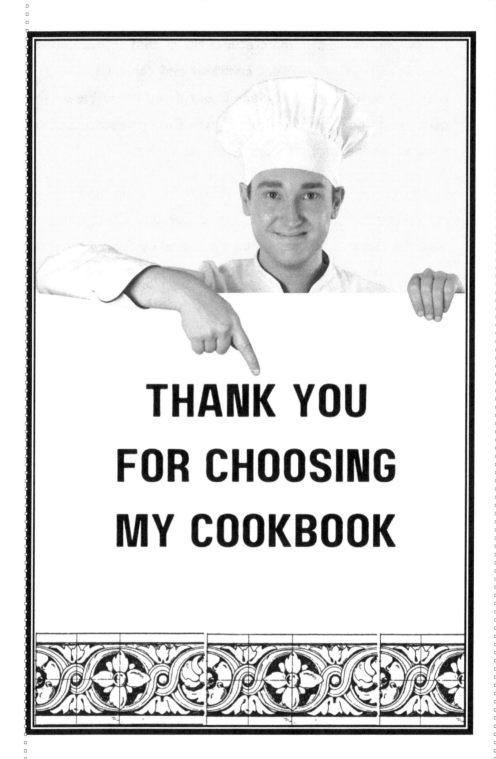

CPSIA information can be obtained
at www.ICGtesting.com
Printed in the USA
BVHW092347080322
630895BV00008B/113